DANIEL FAST DIET

COOKBOOK

A Spiritual Diet Guide to Lose Weight, Eliminate Heart Disease, and Nourish Your Spirit, Soul, and Body

Sarah Hayes, RD

Copyright Page

The recipes and information presented in this cookbook are intended for general informational purposes only. While the author and publisher have made every effort to ensure that the content is accurate and up-to-date, no guarantee is given regarding the completeness, reliability, or suitability of the information provided.

Contents

INTRODUCTION

Embarking on a journey towards better health and spiritual growth often leads us to explore various diets and fasting practices. One such profound and meaningful path is the Daniel Fast Diet. This isn't just any diet; it's a deeply spiritual and holistic approach inspired by the biblical prophet Daniel. More than a regimen for nourishing the body, the Daniel Fast Diet is about nurturing the mind and spirit, creating a harmonious balance that can lead to profound personal transformation.

The roots of the Daniel Fast Diet trace back to an ancient story. In the Bible, Daniel chose to consume only simple, plant-based foods and water as an act of devotion and faith. He abstained from rich foods, wine, and meats, opting instead for vegetables, fruits, and grains. This act of faith was not just about physical sustenance but about spiritual discipline and clarity. Today, many people adopt this practice, seeking the same benefits of physical cleansing and spiritual enlightenment that Daniel experienced centuries ago.

The essence of the Daniel Fast Diet lies in its simplicity and purity. It emphasizes whole, unprocessed foods—fruits, vegetables, whole grains, nuts, seeds, and legumes—while excluding animal products, refined sugars, and artificial additives. The focus is on natural, nutrient-rich foods that support overall health and well-being. This diet isn't just about restriction; it's about embracing a bounty of wholesome, nourishing foods that can revitalize your body from the inside out.

In this introduction to the Daniel Fast Diet, we will delve into the principles and practices that make this diet so unique and impactful. We'll explore the spiritual roots and modern interpretations, providing you with a comprehensive guide to embarking on this journey. Whether you are drawn to the Daniel Fast for its potential health benefits, its spiritual significance, or a combination of both, you will find that this diet offers a pathway to a more vibrant, balanced, and meaningful life.

We'll walk you through the practical aspects of the diet—what to eat, what to avoid, and how to prepare. But more importantly, we'll also delve into the deeper connections between food, faith, and well-being. You'll learn how this ancient practice can fit into contemporary life, providing not just a diet, but a lifestyle that fosters physical health and spiritual growth.

As you read through this book, you'll discover that the Daniel Fast Diet is not just a temporary change but a potential catalyst for lasting transformation.

It's an invitation to slow down, reflect, and reconnect with what truly matters. By the end of this journey, you'll find yourself not just physically rejuvenated but spiritually enriched, ready to embrace a healthier and more fulfilling life.

CHAPTER ONE: WHAT PRECISELY DOES THE DANIEL FAST ENTAIL?

The Daniel Fast is a unique blend of diet and spiritual practice inspired by the biblical figure Daniel. It's not just about the food you eat—it's about nourishing your body and soul. Daniel chose to forgo the rich foods and wine from the king's table, opting instead for vegetables and water. This fast is based on that simple, wholesome approach to eating.

So, what does the Daniel Fast look like in everyday life? You'll be filling your plate with fruits, vegetables, whole grains, nuts, seeds, and legumes. You'll avoid meat, dairy, processed foods, sweeteners, and anything that isn't a whole, plant-based food. Basically, it's all about eating as naturally as possible.

But here's the real beauty of the Daniel Fast: it's as much about your spirit as it is about your body. This fast invites you to slow down and be more mindful of your eating habits. It's a time to reflect, pray, and connect more deeply with your faith. Many people find that the discipline required for the Daniel Fast also strengthens their spiritual life, creating a space for prayer and contemplation.

The simplicity of the Daniel Fast can be incredibly refreshing. In a world full of processed, convenience foods, returning to basics can feel like a detox for your whole being. There are plenty of delicious recipes out there to keep your meals interesting and satisfying. Plus, the focus on whole, unprocessed foods often leads to improved health, clearer skin, and more energy.

In essence, the Daniel Fast is about more than just food. It's a journey towards a healthier, more intentional way of living. It's an opportunity to break free from unhealthy habits and to foster a deeper connection with your faith. Whether you're looking to improve your health, deepen your spirituality, or just try something new, the Daniel

Fast offers a path to a more vibrant and fulfilling life.

The origins in the Bible and the historical background

The Daniel Fast has deep biblical roots and a rich historical background that give it special significance. To truly grasp the essence of the Daniel Fast, it's helpful to dive into its origins and the story behind it.

The fast is inspired by the prophet Daniel, whose story is told in the Old Testament. Daniel was captured and taken to Babylon, where he was selected to serve in the king's court. Despite the temptation of the king's lavish meals, Daniel chose to stick to a simple diet that aligned with his faith and commitment to God.

According to the Bible, Daniel asked to eat only vegetables and drink only water, rejecting the royal delicacies. His choice was driven by a desire to stay true to his religious beliefs, even in a foreign and challenging environment. Daniel's faithfulness paid off, as he was blessed with great health and wisdom, serving as an inspiring example of devotion and self-discipline.

Throughout history, Christians have practiced the Daniel Fast as a way to seek spiritual renewal and a closer relationship with God. It mimics Daniel's devotion by focusing on prayer, reflection, and self-control. Typically, this fast involves eating only fruits, vegetables, whole grains, nuts, and drinking water for a set period, often 21 days, mirroring the duration of Daniel's fasting.

The historical context of the Daniel Fast underscores the importance of dietary choices as an expression of faith and spiritual commitment. For centuries, people have turned to this fast during times of seeking direction, personal growth, or deeper spiritual connections.

Today, the Daniel Fast continues to be a meaningful practice for many, offering a structured way to cleanse the body, clear the mind, and nourish the spirit. It's more than just a diet—it's a journey that honors the legacy of Daniel's story and the historical traditions that have shaped its practice.

By embracing the Daniel Fast, you're not just changing what you eat; you're connecting with a timeless tradition that speaks to faith, discipline, and spiritual growth. It's a personal journey that can lead to profound physical and spiritual benefits, reflecting a deeper commitment to living in harmony with one's beliefs and values.

The reasons individuals opt to adhere to this dietary regimen vary greatly.

People choose to follow the Daniel Fast diet for many heartfelt and personal reasons. One of the main draws is the chance to boost overall health. By focusing on whole, plant-based foods and cutting out processed items, many find they feel better—experiencing improvements in digestion, energy levels, and skin clarity. There's a sense of renewed vitality that comes from eating clean, natural foods.

Beyond the physical benefits, the Daniel Fast often appeals to those seeking spiritual growth. This diet is inspired by the biblical story of Daniel, who chose to eat simple, pure foods as an act of faith and devotion. For many, following this diet is a way to reconnect with their spirituality, providing a time for reflection, prayer, and finding inner peace.

The detoxifying aspect of the Daniel Fast is another reason people are drawn to it. In today's world, where processed foods are so prevalent, taking a break to consume only natural, unprocessed foods can feel refreshing and cleansing. It's like hitting a reset button for your body, helping to eliminate toxins and foster healthier eating habits.

The sense of community that often comes with the Daniel Fast is also a big plus. Many people embark on this journey with their church group or friends, creating a supportive environment where everyone encourages each other. This shared experience can make the fast more meaningful and enjoyable.

Lastly, some people see the Daniel Fast as a personal challenge—a way to break free from unhealthy eating patterns and develop a more mindful relationship with food. It takes commitment and discipline, but the rewards in terms of self-control and a deeper understanding of one's eating habits can be profound.

In summary, people are drawn to the Daniel Fast for a mix of health benefits, spiritual growth, detoxification, community support, and personal challenge. It's a holistic approach to better living, offering a path to greater well-being and self-awareness.

CHAPTER TWO: GRASPING THE ESSENTIALS OF NUTRITION

Navigating your nutritional needs while on the Daniel Fast is like embarking on a culinary adventure with your health as the compass. Picture your plate as a canvas, waiting to be filled with a vibrant array of plant-based goodies that will fuel your body and nourish your soul.

Let's start with the basics: fruits, veggies, whole grains, legumes, nuts, and seeds. These are the rock stars of the Daniel Fast, loaded with all the good stuff your body craves—like vitamins, minerals, and antioxidants. Get creative with your meals, mixing and matching ingredients to keep things exciting and your taste buds happy.

Now, let's talk protein. You might be wondering, "Where's the beef?" Well, it's taking a backseat for now, but fear not! Legumes are here to save the day. Beans, lentils, chickpeas—they're all packed with protein and can be tossed into soups, salads, or stir-fries for a satisfying and nutritious meal.

And what about healthy fats? Avocados, nuts, seeds, and olive oil are your go-to gang when it comes to keeping your brain sharp and your hormones in check. Sprinkle some seeds on your salad, drizzle a little olive oil over your veggies, and snack on some avocado toast for good measure.

Now, let's not forget about calcium. With dairy off the table, it's time to get creative. Load up on leafy greens like kale and spinach, sip on fortified plant-based milks, and toss some tofu into your stir-fry for an extra calcium boost.

Last but not least, listen to your body. If you're feeling a bit low on energy, reach for some whole grains or a piece of fruit to give yourself a little pick-me-up. And don't forget to stay hydrated!

Water, herbal teas, infused waters—whatever floats your boat, just keep that hydration flowing.

So there you have it—your roadmap to rocking the Daniel Fast like a pro. Get creative, listen to your body, and most importantly, enjoy the journey to better health and well-being.

Essential Nutrients for Your Body During the Fast

Alright, let's get real about what your body craves during the Daniel Fast! Think of it as a time to give your body the VIP treatment—nourishment that fuels you inside and out.

First off, hydration is your bestie. Keep that water bottle handy and sip on herbal teas to jazz things up a bit. Trust me, your body will thank you for it!

Now, onto protein—because we all want those muscles to stay strong, right? Luckily, there are plenty of plant-based options like beans, lentils, nuts, seeds, and tofu that pack a punch in the protein department. Get creative and toss them into salads, stir-fries, or whip up a hearty bean chili.

Carbs, anyone? Yes, please! But we're talking about the good stuff—whole grains like brown rice, quinoa, and oats that keep your energy levels steady and your tummy satisfied. Plus, they're delicious and versatile, so you'll never get bored.

Fruits and veggies are where it's at for vitamins, minerals, and all-around goodness. Load up your plate with colorful produce to give your body the nutrients it craves and keep your immune system in tip-top shape.

Last but not least, let's talk about fats. We're talking about the healthy kind—avocados, nuts, seeds, and olive oil—that keep your heart happy and your skin glowing. So go ahead, drizzle some olive oil on your salad or snack on some avocado toast guilt-free.

Bottom line: Listen to your body, have fun experimenting with new flavors, and remember that taking care of yourself is what it's all about during the Daniel Fast. You got this!

Achieving the Right Balance of Proteins, Carbs, and Fats

Navigating the world of balancing proteins, carbs, and fats on the Daniel Fast can seem daunting at first, but fear not! With a little guidance and creativity, you can easily achieve a well-rounded diet that supports your health goals while following the principles of this spiritual journey.

Firstly, let's talk about proteins. While meat is off the table during the Daniel Fast, there are plenty of plant-based protein sources to choose from. Think lentils, beans, chickpeas, quinoa, tofu, tempeh, and nuts. Incorporating these into your meals ensures you're getting the protein your body needs to thrive.

Now, onto carbs. Carbohydrates are your body's primary source of energy, so it's essential to include them in your meals. Opt for complex carbohydrates like whole grains (brown rice, oats, barley), fruits, and vegetables. These provide sustained energy and essential nutrients to keep you feeling full and satisfied throughout the day.

Lastly, fats play a crucial role in your diet, providing energy, supporting cell growth, and aiding in nutrient absorption. Focus on healthy fats like avocados, nuts, seeds, and olive oil. These fats are rich in omega-3 fatty acids and are excellent for heart health and overall well-being.

Balancing these macronutrients doesn't have to be complicated. Start by building your meals around a variety of plant-based proteins, complemented by wholesome carbs and healthy fats. Get creative in the kitchen with flavorful herbs, spices, and sauces to add depth and excitement to your meals.

Remember, the key is to listen to your body and honor its needs while on this journey. Pay attention to how different foods make you feel and adjust your meals accordingly. With a little planning and a lot of delicious plant-based ingredients, you can easily strike the perfect balance of proteins, carbs, and fats on the Daniel Fast, nourishing your body, mind, and spirit along the way.

CHAPTER THREE: HOW IT WORKS: RULES AND FOUNDATIONS

Picture this: you're not just changing your meals, you're reshaping your relationship with food and spirituality.

The heart of the Daniel Fast lies in what you put on your plate. Think lots of colorful fruits and veggies, hearty grains, nuts, and legumes—all the good stuff straight from the earth. And on the flip side, it's a farewell to things like meat, dairy, sugar, and anything that's been too processed. But here's the kicker: it's not just about what you eat, it's about why.

See, the Daniel Fast is all about intention. It's about taking a pause in your day to make mindful choices that nourish your body, respect the planet, and maybe even bring you closer to your faith. Whether you're in it for the health benefits, the ethical reasons, or the spiritual journey, the Daniel Fast is your chance to walk the walk and live your values.

Now, let's talk about the journey itself. It's not always easy. There might be cravings, moments of doubt, or days when you just miss your usual go-tos. But here's the beautiful part: every challenge is a chance to grow. It's a chance to push past your comfort zone, to discover new flavors and recipes, and to connect with something deeper within yourself.

And the best part? The rewards are real. We're talking more energy, clearer thinking, and a sense of purpose that goes way beyond what's on your plate. So, whether you're just starting out or you've been on this journey for a while, remember this: the Daniel Fast isn't just a diet, it's a way of living — a way to nourish your body, feed your soul, and maybe even change the world, one meal at a time.

Foods You Can Eat

So, what's on the menu during the Daniel Fast? Well, you might be surprised by the variety of tasty treats you can enjoy while sticking to the plan. Here's a peek at some of the yummy options that'll keep you satisfied and smiling:

Fruit Frenzy: Get ready to dive into a fruity paradise! Whether you're munching on juicy apples, succulent berries, zesty oranges, or creamy bananas, there's a whole world of flavor waiting for you. Plus, they're not just delicious—they're packed with all sorts of good stuff to keep you feeling your best.

Veggie Delight: Say hello to your new best friends: veggies! From crispy carrots to crunchy bell peppers, leafy greens to savory squash, the veggie aisle is your playground. And the best part?

They're bursting with vitamins and nutrients to keep your body humming along nicely.

Grain Train: All aboard the grain train! Brown rice, quinoa, oats—take your pick! These hearty grains are the perfect foundation for a satisfying meal. Packed with fiber and complex carbs, they'll keep you feeling full and fueled up for whatever the day throws your way.

Legume Love: Beans, lentils, chickpeas—oh my! These little guys are true superheroes in the kitchen. Packed with protein, fiber, and all sorts of essential nutrients, they're a must-have for any Daniel Fast meal. Whether you're whipping up a hearty stew or a zesty salad, legumes are sure to steal the show.

Nutty Goodness: Need a snack? Nuts and seeds to the rescue! Whether you're munching on almonds, walnuts, chia seeds, or flaxseeds, these crunchy treats are the perfect pick-me-up. Sprinkle them on your morning oatmeal, toss them in a salad, or just enjoy them by the handful—they're delicious any way you slice it.

Plant-Powered Protein: Who needs meat when you've got tofu, tempeh, and edamame? These plant-based powerhouses are packed with protein and flavor, making them the perfect addition to any meal. Whether you're stir-frying, grilling, or sautéing, these versatile ingredients are sure to hit the spot.

Spice it Up: Last but not least, don't forget to add a little flair to your meals with herbs and spices. Whether you're a fan of fiery chili flakes, zesty garlic, or aromatic basil, there's no shortage of ways to jazz up your dishes and make them sing.

So there you have it—eating on the Daniel Fast is anything but boring! With so many delicious options to choose from, you'll be well on your way to health and happiness in no time. Bon appétit!

Foods to Steer Clear Of

When you're diving into the Daniel Fast, it's like embarking on a journey where you're mindful of every bite you take. So, what's off the table during this adventure? Well, think of it this way: anything overly processed or refined, like those tempting sugary treats or that bag of chips calling your name from the vending machine—best to give those a pass.

Then there's the meat and dairy aisle. Yep, they're a no-go zone too. It might seem like a big shift at first, especially if you're used to a burger or a cheesy pizza, but trust me, you'll find plenty of delicious plant-based alternatives to satisfy your cravings.

Oh, and say farewell to your morning coffee or evening glass of wine—at least for now. During the Daniel Fast, we're opting for herbal teas and lots of water to keep us hydrated and feeling good.

Remember, the goal here is to embrace foods that are as close to nature as possible, packed with all the good stuff your body needs. So, as you navigate your way through the Daniel Fast, keep that in mind, and you'll be on the right track to nourishing both your body and your soul.

CHAPTER FOUR: STRATEGIES FOR ORGANIZING YOUR MEALS

Planning meals for the Daniel Fast can seem a bit daunting at first, but with some creativity and preparation, it can be a rewarding experience. Here are some friendly, down-to-earth tips to help you navigate meal planning on the Daniel Fast:

1. Start with a Plan:

- Before you even think about grocery shopping, take a moment to plan out your meals for the week. Look up some Daniel Fast-friendly recipes that excite you and write down a plan for breakfast, lunch, dinner, and snacks.

- Making a detailed shopping list is a lifesaver. It ensures you have all the ingredients you need, keeps you organized, and helps you avoid the temptation of non-compliant foods.

2. Keep it Simple:

- Don't stress about making elaborate meals every day. Simple can be delicious! Focus on whole foods and straightforward recipes.

- Think about hearty salads with lots of veggies, easy vegetable stir-fries, and grain bowls with a variety of toppings. Sometimes, the simplest meals are the most satisfying.

3. Stock Up on Staples:

- Make sure your pantry is well-stocked with essentials like quinoa, brown rice, beans, lentils, nuts, seeds, and whole grains. These ingredients are incredibly versatile and can be mixed and matched in countless ways.

- Don't forget frozen fruits and veggies. They're just as nutritious as fresh ones and super convenient for quick meals.

4. Get Creative with Flavors:

- Limiting certain ingredients doesn't mean your meals have to be boring. Play around with different herbs, spices, and natural flavorings to keep things interesting.

- Use garlic, ginger, cumin, turmeric, paprika, and fresh herbs like cilantro and parsley. Natural enhancers like lemon juice, lime juice, and vinegar can really make your dishes pop.

5. Embrace Plant-Based Proteins:

- Protein is crucial, and on the Daniel Fast, you'll need to think outside the box. Include tofu, tempeh, chickpeas, black beans, lentils, and edamame in your meals to ensure you're getting enough protein.

- Nuts and seeds are also great for adding a protein boost. Try sprinkling chia seeds or hemp seeds on salads or smoothie bowls.

6. Plan for Snacks:

- Healthy snacks are your best friend during the Daniel Fast. Keep a variety of fruits, raw veggies, nuts, and homemade energy bars or granola within reach for when you need a quick bite.

- Prep your snacks in advance and portion them out so they're ready to grab and go. This helps you avoid reaching for less healthy options.

7. Prep Ahead:

- Spend some time prepping ingredients ahead of time. Chop vegetables, cook grains and beans, and portion out ingredients so they're ready to go when you need them.

- Batch cooking can be a game-changer. Make large portions of your favorite dishes that you can eat throughout the week. Soups, stews, and casseroles are perfect for this.

8. Stay Flexible:

- Remember, meal planning is here to make your life easier, not stress you out. Don't be afraid to mix things up and try new recipes. And if you stray from your plan occasionally, that's okay!

- The key is to listen to your body and nourish it with wholesome foods. If you find a recipe or ingredient you love, don't hesitate to repeat it.

9. Explore New Recipes:

- Use the Daniel Fast as a chance to try new recipes and cuisines. Explore dishes from different cultures that fit the guidelines of the fast.

- Experiment with new cooking techniques. Try roasting vegetables, making homemade sauces, or even fermenting foods like sauerkraut.

10. Connect with a Community:

- It can be really helpful to connect with others who are also following the Daniel Fast. Join online forums, social media groups, or local communities to share tips, recipes, and support.

- Sharing your experiences and challenges with others can provide encouragement and new ideas to keep your meal planning fresh and exciting.

By following these tips, you'll find that planning your meals on the Daniel Fast can be a fun and enriching experience. It's a chance to explore new foods, develop healthier eating habits, and deepen your spiritual practice, all while enjoying a variety of delicious and nutritious meals.

Preparing for the Fast

It can feel like a big step, but it's an exciting journey that can bring wonderful changes to your health and spiritual life. Here are some tips to help you prepare and make the most of this meaningful experience:

1. Know Your Why: The Daniel Fast is more than just changing what you eat. Think about why you're doing it. Are you seeking spiritual growth, better health, or a fresh start? Understanding your motivation can keep you inspired and focused throughout the fast.

2. Plan Ahead: Switching to a plant-based diet can be tough without a plan. Look up some tasty recipes, make a shopping list, and fill your pantry with whole grains, fruits, vegetables, nuts, and legumes. Having delicious, nutritious foods on hand will make it easier to stick to your plan.

3. Set Realistic Goals: Be clear about what you hope to achieve. Maybe you want to feel more connected spiritually, improve your health, or clear your mind. Set achievable goals to keep yourself motivated. Remember, it's about progress, not perfection.

4. Prepare Your Mind and Spirit: The Daniel Fast isn't just about your body; it's about your whole self. Spend some time in prayer, meditation, or journaling to prepare mentally and spiritually. This can help you stay centered and focused.

5. Find a Support Buddy: Everything's easier with a friend. Do the fast with a friend, family member, or group. Share recipes, encourage each other, and talk about your experiences. Having someone to share the journey with makes it more enjoyable.

6. Be Kind to Yourself: It's normal to face challenges and cravings, especially at the beginning. Don't be hard on yourself. If you slip

up, it's okay—just refocus and keep going. Every small step forward is progress.

7. Stay Hydrated: Drinking plenty of water is crucial. It helps your body detox and function well. Try herbal teas or water with a splash of lemon for variety.

8. Enjoy the Process: This is a chance to discover new foods and recipes. Enjoy the journey and celebrate the small victories and changes you notice along the way.

Getting ready for the Daniel Fast is about more than changing your diet. It's about preparing for a transformative experience that can benefit your body, mind, and spirit. By taking these steps, you'll be ready to start this journey with confidence and purpose, opening yourself up to all the benefits it can bring.

Getting Your Mind and Spirit Ready

Starting the Daniel Fast is about more than just changing your diet; it's about getting your mind and spirit ready for a meaningful journey. This fast is a chance to nourish not just your body, but also your soul and your mental well-being. Here are some steps to help you prepare in a way that feels natural and supportive.

Setting the Right Mindset

First, get into the right mindset. The Daniel Fast is a commitment, and understanding your reasons for doing it can make all the difference. Take some time to think about why you're choosing this path. Are you looking to improve your health, deepen your spiritual life, or both? Write down your reasons and goals. This can be a helpful reminder when things get tough and keep you focused on your purpose.

Nourishing Your Spirit

Spiritually, get ready to engage more deeply with your faith or personal beliefs. You might want to incorporate more prayer, meditation, or reading of inspirational texts into your daily routine. Starting and ending your day with a moment of reflection can be grounding. If you're part of a faith community, lean on them for support. Sharing this journey with others can provide encouragement and a sense of connection.

Emotional Preparation

Emotionally, prepare for a range of feelings. Changing your diet and routine can be challenging, and it's okay to feel frustrated or tempted at times. Be kind to yourself and recognize that it's all part of the process. Keeping a journal can be a great way to process your thoughts and track your progress. Write about your experiences, your struggles, and your victories, no matter how small they might seem.

Practical Steps

On a practical level, planning ahead can make the transition smoother. Make a list of foods you can eat during the fast and find some recipes that you're excited to try. This isn't just about cutting out foods; it's an opportunity to explore new, wholesome ingredients that can be both delicious and nourishing. Preparing meals in advance can save you time and reduce the stress of daily cooking, giving you more space to focus on the spiritual aspects of the fast.

Building a Supportive Environment

Creating a supportive environment is crucial. Let your friends and family know about your decision to undertake the Daniel Fast. Their understanding and support can be incredibly helpful, especially if you find yourself struggling. Having people who cheer you on can make a big difference.

In summary, preparing your mind and spirit for the Daniel Fast is about combining practical steps with personal reflection and spiritual practice. By setting clear intentions, embracing spiritual rituals, acknowledging your emotional journey, and planning ahead, you set yourself up for a successful and transformative experience. Remember, this is a personal journey towards better health and deeper connection, and every step you take is a move towards a more vibrant, fulfilling life.

CHAPTER FIVE: ESTABLISHING PERSONAL OBJECTIVES AND ASPIRATIONS

Setting personal goals and intentions on the Daniel Fast is an enriching practice that can profoundly enhance your experience and help you derive maximum benefit from this period of dietary and spiritual discipline. By taking the time to identify and articulate your aspirations, you not only imbue your fast with purpose and direction but also lay the groundwork for meaningful personal growth and transformation.

Begin by engaging in introspection and reflection to discern what you hope to achieve through the Daniel Fast. Are you primarily seeking physical improvements, such as enhanced health, increased energy, or weight management? Or perhaps your goals are more spiritually oriented, centered around deepening your connection to your faith, cultivating inner peace, or gaining clarity on your life's purpose. Maybe you're aiming to foster greater mindfulness and gratitude in your daily life, or to strengthen your self-discipline and resilience. Whatever your intentions, expressing them clearly and specifically can provide a powerful focal point for your journey and serve as a source of motivation and accountability.

Once you've identified your overarching goals, consider breaking them down into smaller, actionable steps that you can incorporate into your daily routine. For example, if your aim is to improve your physical health, you might set objectives related to exercise, hydration, or meal planning. This could involve committing to a regular workout regimen, drinking a certain amount of water each day, or experimenting with new plant-based recipes to keep your meals interesting and nutritious. If your focus is more on spiritual growth, you might establish goals related to prayer, meditation, scripture study, or acts of service. This could entail setting aside dedicated time each day for spiritual practices, participating in a study group or discussion forum, or volunteering in your community to support those in need. If mindfulness is a priority for you, you might set goals around practices like journaling, deep breathing, or mindfulness exercises. This could involve keeping a gratitude journal to record daily blessings, practicing mindfulness meditation to cultivate present-moment awareness, or engaging in relaxation techniques to reduce stress and promote emotional well-being.

As you embark on your Daniel Fast journey, keep in mind that your goals and intentions may evolve over time, and that's perfectly okay. Be open to the insights and revelations that emerge along the way, and allow yourself the flexibility to adapt your goals as needed in response to changing circumstances or inner guidance. Remember that the Daniel Fast is not just about what you eat—it's about nourishing your body, mind, and spirit in holistic harmony. By setting personal goals and intentions that resonate with your deepest desires and values, you can infuse your fast with purpose and meaning, and experience profound growth and transformation that extends far beyond the duration of the fast itself. Embrace this sacred time as an opportunity for self-discovery, renewal, and empowerment, and trust that the seeds you plant during this season will yield abundant fruit in the days and weeks to come.

Maintaining Your Energy Levels Throughout the Day

1. Start Your Day Right: Breakfast sets the tone for the rest of the day, so make sure it's packed with nutrients to fuel your body. Consider adding variety to your morning meals by experimenting

with different grains, fruits, nuts, and seeds. For example, try a hearty bowl of overnight oats topped with sliced bananas, almonds, and a drizzle of almond butter for a satisfying start.

2. Hydrate, Hydrate, Hydrate: Proper hydration is essential for maintaining energy levels and supporting overall health. While water is the best choice for staying hydrated, you can mix things up by incorporating herbal teas or infused water with slices of cucumber, lemon, or mint for added flavor and hydration benefits.

3. Strategic Snacking: When hunger strikes between meals, reach for snacks that provide a

balance of carbohydrates, protein, and healthy fats to keep your energy levels steady. Consider options like apple slices with almond butter, a handful of trail mix, or whole grain crackers with avocado to keep you feeling satisfied until your next meal.

4. Protein Power: Including protein-rich foods in your meals is essential for sustaining energy levels and supporting muscle repair and growth. Incorporate plant-based protein sources such as beans, lentils, chickpeas, tofu, and edamame into your meals to ensure you're getting an adequate intake of this vital nutrient.

5. Mindful Meal Timing: Aim to eat regular meals throughout the day to keep your energy levels stable and prevent dips in blood sugar. Skipping meals or going too long between meals can lead to fatigue and cravings, so prioritize consistent meal timing to keep your energy levels steady.

6. Complex Carbohydrates for Sustained Energy: Choose complex carbohydrates such as whole grains, legumes, and starchy vegetables over simple carbohydrates like refined grains and sugars. Complex carbs provide a steady source of energy and are rich in fiber, which helps keep you feeling full and satisfied.

7. The Power of Plants: Embrace the abundance of plant-based foods available on the Daniel Fast to nourish your body and support your energy needs. Fill your plate with a colorful array of fruits, vegetables, whole grains, nuts, seeds, and legumes to ensure you're getting a wide variety of nutrients to support optimal energy levels and overall health.

8. Prioritize Rest and Recovery: In addition to nourishing your body with wholesome foods, prioritize rest and recovery to support energy levels and overall well-being. Aim for 7-9 hours of quality sleep each night, and incorporate relaxation techniques such as meditation, yoga, or deep breathing exercises to help manage stress and promote relaxation.

By incorporating these human-friendly strategies into your daily routine, you can support steady energy levels throughout the day while nourishing your body with nutrient-rich, plant-based foods on the Daniel Fast.

Crafting Your List for the Grocery Store

When it comes to crafting your grocery shopping list for the Daniel Fast, think of it as a chance to get creative and nourish both your body and spirit. Start by focusing on whole, plant-based foods that are in line with the principles of the fast.

First, load up on fresh fruits and vegetables. Think colorful salads bursting with leafy greens, vibrant bell peppers, crunchy carrots, and juicy tomatoes. Stock up on a variety of fruits like apples, bananas, berries, and citrus fruits to satisfy your sweet cravings and provide essential nutrients.

Next, explore the world of whole grains and legumes. Fill your cart with hearty staples like brown rice, quinoa, lentils, and beans. These nutrient-dense foods will keep you feeling satisfied and energized throughout the fast.

Don't forget about healthy fats and protein sources. Add avocados, nuts, seeds, and tofu to your list for a boost of omega-3s and plant-based protein. These ingredients will add flavor and depth to your meals while supporting your overall health.

Finally, round out your shopping list with pantry essentials like herbs, spices, and plant-based condiments. Get creative with flavors by experimenting with different seasonings and sauces to elevate your dishes without compromising the integrity of the fast.

As you navigate the aisles, remember to stay mindful of your choices and their alignment with the principles of the Daniel Fast. By prioritizing whole, plant-based foods and avoiding processed items, you'll not only nourish your body but also honor the spiritual journey you're on. Happy shopping and happy fasting!

CHAPTER SIX: OVERCOMING CHALLENGES ON DANIEL FAST DIET

Navigating the ups and downs of the Daniel Fast journey can feel like a rollercoaster ride at times, but overcoming challenges is all part of the experience. Whether you're battling cravings for your favorite comfort foods or struggling to find satisfying meal options, rest assured, you're not alone.

One of the biggest hurdles many face is adjusting to the limited food choices allowed on the Daniel Fast. Saying goodbye to beloved staples like dairy, meat, and processed foods can be tough, especially in the beginning. But with a bit of creativity and resourcefulness, you'll discover a world of delicious, plant-based alternatives that not only satisfy your taste buds but also nourish your body.

Another common challenge is dealing with social situations where your dietary restrictions may feel like a burden or an inconvenience. Whether it's attending a family gathering or dining out with friends, explaining your dietary choices to others can be daunting. But remember, your health and well-being are worth prioritizing, and those who care about you will likely be supportive once they understand your reasons for following the Daniel Fast.

Then there's the emotional aspect of the journey. It's normal to experience moments of frustration, temptation, or doubt along the way. Remembering your reasons for embarking on this path—whether it's to improve your health, deepen your faith, or simply challenge yourself—can help keep you motivated and focused during those tough times.

Ultimately, overcoming challenges on the Daniel Fast is not just about enduring hardships but also about embracing growth and transformation. Each obstacle you face is an opportunity to learn more about yourself, strengthen your resolve, and deepen your connection to your goals and values. So take it one day at a time, lean on your support network, and celebrate every small victory along the way. You've got this!

Managing Cravings: Tips and Techniques

Handling cravings during the Daniel Fast can sometimes feel like wrestling with your own desires, but there are some tricks to help you stay strong and on track.

First off, it's crucial to understand what's behind those cravings. Are you genuinely hungry, or is it more of an emotional or habitual urge? Once you've figured that out, you can tackle it head-on. If it's hunger, make sure your meals are filling and balanced, with plenty of plant-based protein, fiber, and healthy fats to keep you satisfied.

When those cravings hit hard, distraction can be your best friend. Dive into activities that keep your mind and hands busy, whether it's taking a stroll, diving into a hobby, or having a heart-to-heart with a friend. Sometimes, just shifting your focus away from food can make those cravings fade away.

It's also a smart move to have some healthy snacks on standby. Stock up on fruits, veggies, nuts, and seeds so you can nibble on something nutritious when the cravings come knocking. These snacks not only curb hunger but also fit perfectly with the Daniel Fast guidelines.

And don't forget to stay hydrated! Sometimes, what feels like hunger is really just thirst in disguise. Keep a water bottle handy and sip throughout the day. Herbal teas or infused water can add some flavor and variety to your hydration game.

Above all, be kind to yourself. Cravings are a normal part of making any dietary change, and it's okay to slip up now and then. If you find yourself giving in, don't beat yourself up. Just acknowledge it, learn from it, and get back on track. You've got this!

Managing Social Occasions and Gatherings

Navigating social events and gatherings while sticking to the Daniel Fast can feel like a bit of a balancing act. You want to honor your commitment to your health and spirituality, but you also don't want to miss out on the fun and connection that comes with socializing. Here are some down-to-earth tips to help you handle these situations like a pro:

1. Plan with Purpose: Take a peek at the menu or have a chat with the host beforehand. This way, you can mentally prepare and even offer to whip up a Daniel Fast-friendly dish to share.

2. Open Up: Don't be shy about sharing your dietary choices with your pals or family. Most folks are pretty understanding and might even be curious to try some of your Daniel Fast recipes.

3. Prioritize People: Keep in mind that gatherings are about more than just food. Focus on enjoying the company of your loved ones and diving into good conversations rather than fixating on what's on the menu.

4. Flexibility is Key: While it's important to stick to your Daniel Fast guidelines, it's also okay to be a bit flexible when necessary. If options are limited,

aim for the healthiest choices available without stressing too much.

5. BYOS (Bring Your Own Snacks): If you're unsure about the food situation, bring along some Daniel Fast-friendly snacks or dishes to share. This ensures you'll have something to munch on and gives others a chance to try something new.

6. Keep the Vibes Positive: Lastly, maintain a positive attitude throughout the event. Remind yourself why you're following the Daniel Fast and focus on the positive impacts it's having on your health and spiritual journey.

Approaching social gatherings with a mix of mindfulness, communication, and a willingness to roll with the punches will help you navigate them like a champ while staying true to your commitment to the Daniel Fast.

CHAPTER SEVEN: NAVIGATING LIFE AFTER THE FAST

Transitioning after completing the Daniel Fast is like coming back down to earth after a spiritual and nutritional high. It's all about finding your footing again while staying true to the principles that guided you through the fast.

So, where do you start? Well, it's all about taking it slow and steady. Listen to your body—it's got plenty to say after all those days of clean eating. Start by reintroducing simple, wholesome foods like fruits, veggies, and whole grains. Think of it as giving your body a gentle nudge back into the rhythm of regular eating without overwhelming it.

And hey, don't forget the plant-based vibe! Those fruits and veggies aren't just good for you; they're in line with the whole spirit of the Daniel Fast. Plus, they're packed with all the good stuff your body needs to keep feeling awesome.

But transitioning after the fast isn't just about what you eat—it's about staying connected to the deeper meaning behind it all. Take some time to reflect on your journey, maybe journal a bit or spend a moment in quiet gratitude. And if prayer or meditation is your thing, now's the perfect time to dive back in.

Lastly, be kind to yourself. Transitioning back to "normal" eating might come with a few bumps in the road, and that's okay. Give yourself permission to take it one day at a time, and remember that the goal is to create a lifestyle that's as nourishing for your soul as it is for your body.

Maintaining Motivation and Staying Focused

Staying motivated and on track during the Daniel Fast can feel like a rollercoaster ride of ups and downs, but trust me, it's totally doable with the right approach. Picture this: you've got your goals front and center, reminding yourself why you started this journey in the first place. Whether it's about feeling healthier, getting closer to your spirituality, or simply trying out something new, keeping your 'why' in focus can be your secret weapon to staying on track.

Now, let's talk about having your squad behind you. Whether it's your family, friends, or a supportive online community, having people who get what you're going through can be a game-changer. Sharing your wins and struggles with others not only keeps you accountable but also pumps you up with encouragement and inspiration.

Oh, and speaking of being prepared, that's key too. Stock up your kitchen with loads of tasty, Daniel Fast-approved foods, and have some easy-peasy recipes up your sleeve for those moments when hunger strikes out of nowhere. And hey, don't be afraid to get creative in the kitchen. Trying out new flavors and dishes can make this whole journey way more exciting.

Now, let's get real for a sec. We're all human, and slip-ups are bound to happen. But guess what? That's totally okay! Instead of beating yourself up over a little stumble, use it as a chance to learn and grow. Remember, progress is progress, no matter how small. So, celebrate those wins, keep that positive vibe going, and before you know it, you'll be cruising through your Daniel Fast journey like a pro.

Sustaining Your Fresh Healthy Routines

So, you've taken the plunge into the Daniel Fast and embraced a healthier lifestyle. That's awesome! But let's be real—keeping up with these changes isn't always a walk in the park. Here are some down-to-earth tips to help you stay on track during the fast:

First off, cut yourself some slack. Nobody's perfect, and slip-ups happen. Instead of beating yourself up about it, use slip-ups as learning experiences. Every step forward, no matter how small, is progress.

Meal prep is your best friend. Seriously. Take some time each week to plan out your meals and snacks. Having healthy options at your fingertips makes it a whole lot easier to resist the urge to dive headfirst into a bag of chips or cookies.

And speaking of support, don't go it alone. Rally the troops—whether it's your best friend, your partner, or your mom—and let them know what you're up to. Having someone in your corner to cheer you on can make all the difference when the going gets tough.

Listen to your body. It's trying to tell you something. Pay attention to hunger cues and cravings, and fuel up with nutritious foods that make you feel good inside and out.

And last but definitely not least, be kind to yourself. This journey isn't always easy, but you're doing it for a reason. Celebrate your wins, no matter how small, and give yourself a pat on the back for showing up and putting in the effort.

With a little bit of commitment, planning, support, and self-love, you can totally crush it on the Daniel Fast. You've got this!

CHAPTER EIGHT: DELECTABLE RECIPE IDEAS AND SUGGESTIONS YOU MUST TRY

DELECTABLE BREAKFAST IDEAS

Southwestern Potato Bowl

<u>Ingredients Needed</u>

4 large Yukon Gold potatoes, scrubbed

1 (15-ounce) can pinto beans, drained, rinsed, and mashed

½ to 1 cup Ro-Tel Diced Tomatoes and Green Chilies (look for no- or low-salt versions)

8 ounces frozen corn (we prefer white corn as it is sweeter!)

1 red bell pepper, diced

2 scallions (white and green parts), chopped

2 to 4 cups fresh spinach

Fresh cilantro, for garnish

Hot sauce

Method

Prepare the Yukon Gold potatoes any way you prefer: Microwave the potatoes, two at a time, for 8 to 10 minutes, or until each potato is cooked through. Or preheat the oven to 375°F. Place the potatoes directly on the oven rack. Bake for 45 minutes to 1 hour, or until cooked through.

Place the beans in a microwavable bowl and heat for 60 seconds. Or, if you prefer to use the stovetop, place the beans in a small pot over medium-high heat, stirring occasionally, for about 2 minutes, or until thoroughly warmed. With the backside of a fork, smash about half of the beans. Add the desired amount of Ro-Tel tomatoes to the beans, along with the corn, pepper, and green onion. Set aside.

In the base of 4 serving bowls, place a layer of fresh spinach, followed by a potato, cut in half or cubed (your choice). Add the bean mixture on top of the potato and garnish with cilantro and a few shakes of your favorite hot sauce. Don't forget to serve along with a green salad or a heaping helping of cooked greens.

Aloo Baingan

<u>**Ingredients Needed**</u>

1 medium purple eggplant, unpeeled and cut into ½-inch cubes

5 medium potatoes, peeled and cut into ½-inch cubes

1 teaspoon grated ginger

1 small jalapeño, seeded and chopped

1 tablespoon coriander powder

½ teaspoon paprika

½ teaspoon turmeric

1 teaspoon cumin seed

Pinch of asafoetida (hing) (optional)

1 medium tomato, cut into ½-inch cubes

1½ cups fat-free tomato sauce

½ to 1 teaspoon salt (optional)

2 tablespoons chopped cilantro

Method

Preheat the oven to 400°F. Lay out chopped eggplant on one non-stick cooking sheet and chopped potato on the other. Roast eggplant for approximately 15 minutes, until it is starting to soften but not mushy. Roast potatoes for approximately 25 minutes, until edges are starting to brown and potatoes are just cooked.

While eggplant and potatoes are roasting, place the grated ginger, jalapeño, coriander powder, paprika, turmeric, and 2 tablespoons of water in a small bowl. Mix to make a paste.

Heat a cast iron or nonstick pot over medium heat. Test the heat by adding one cumin seed to the pot; if seed cracks right away, the pot is heated to the right temperature.

Add cumin seeds and asafoetida after seed cracks. Add the spice mixture and stir-fry for 20 seconds, stirring continuously.

Add chopped tomato and stir-fry for a minute. Add tomato sauce. Mix well.

Add roasted potatoes and eggplant. Mix gently and let it simmer for 3 to 4 minutes on medium-low heat. Taste and add salt, if needed. Turn off the heat and add chopped cilantro. Mix well.

Chef's Note: Asafoetida is a spice derived from the resin extracted from a plant root. It has a pungent aroma that is very strong when raw but works as a flavor enhancer when cooked. It gives a unique flavor to most Indian dishes. It is also called "Hing," available in most Indian grocery stores.

Herbed Fingerling Potatoes

<u>Ingredients Needed</u>

1 ½ pounds fingerling potatoes, scrubbed

1 cup vegetable broth

1 tablespoon fresh marjoram

1 tablespoon fresh thyme

1 teaspoon fresh rosemary

1 teaspoon onion flakes

1 teaspoon garlic powder

sea salt

ground black pepper

1 tablespoon fresh chives

Method

Add the potatoes to a saucepot and fill with enough water to cover the potatoes. Bring to a boil and cook on medium-high heat, covered, for 20 minutes until the potatoes are tender when poked with a fork.

In the meanwhile, place the broth, marjoram, thyme, rosemary, onion flakes, and garlic powder in a saucepan. Mix well and let stand until the potatoes are ready.

Drain the potatoes and run under cold water until cool enough to handle. Cut them lengthwise into halves.

Bring the broth to a boil, add the potatoes, stir well, and cook for about 5 minutes on medium-high heat, stirring occasionally, until the broth is absorbed by the potatoes.

Sprinkle with salt, pepper, and chives and serve warm.

Apple, Grapefruit, Pomegranate Salad

Ingredients Needed

1 apple, cut into medium dice

1 grapefruit, cut into segments

1 pomegranate, seeded

1 tablespoon lemon juice (optional)

sea salt

freshly ground black pepper

1 tablespoon fresh mint leaves, roughly chopped

2 cups baby romaine lettuce

Method

Place the apple, grapefruit, and pomegranate seeds in a bowl. Add the lemon juice (if using), salt, and pepper and mix well.

Garnish with fresh mint and serve on a bed of greens

Fava Bean Salad

Ingredients Needed

4 cups cooked fava beans, or two 15-ounce cans, drained and rinsed

2 large tomatoes, chopped

4 scallions (white and green parts), sliced

1 large cucumber, peeled, halved, seeded, and diced

½ cup finely chopped cilantro

1 jalapeño pepper, minced (for less heat, remove the seeds)

Zest of 1 lemon and juice of 2 lemons

2 cloves garlic, peeled and minced

1 teaspoon cumin seeds, toasted and ground

Salt and freshly ground black pepper to taste

Method

Combine all ingredients in a large bowl and mix well. Chill for 1 hour before serving.

Green Bean and Mango Salad

Ingredients Needed

FOR SALAD:

3 cups green beans or Asian long beans

2 slightly underripe mangos

1 cup cherry or grape tomatoes, halved

¼ cup fresh cilantro

3 green onions, sliced

¼ cup peanuts, crushed

FOR DRESSING:

2 tablespoons fresh lime juice

1 tablespoon gluten-free tamari

½ teaspoon unrefined cane sugar

1 fresh Thai chili, minced (optional)

Method

Bring a pan of water to a boil. Add the green beans and cook for up to 2 minutes, until bright green and tender-crisp. Drain, then plunge them into a bowl of ice water to halt the cooking process. Drain again. Trim the ends and slice the beans in half lengthwise. Place them in a large bowl and set aside.

Seed and peel the mango and slice into long, thin strips. Add mango to the green beans, along with the tomatoes, cilantro, onion, and peanuts.

Whisk together the lime juice, tamari, cane sugar, and chili in a small bowl. Pour over the salad, toss, and serve. The salad can be made and dressed ahead of time and left to chill and marinate in the fridge for up to 3 hours.

"Nacho" Vegan Baked Potato

Ingredients Needed

1 large baking potato

1½ teaspoons nutritional yeast (optional)

½ cup black beans, either canned or prepared as directed for Black Beans

¼ cup salsa of your choice

¼ to ½ avocado, cubed, sliced, or smashed

Salt and black pepper to taste

Cilantro for garnish

Lime wedges for garnish

Method

Preheat the oven to 450°F (230°C) if baking the potato (rather than microwaving it).

Pierce the potato with a fork or knife a few times to allow the steam to escape. Bake in the oven for about 40 minutes, or microwave for 4 to 6 minutes, depending on the size of the potato. Pierce the potato with a fork or knife to check if it is soft and cooked through.

When the potato is done, slice it open, and sprinkle on the nutritional yeast, if using.

Layer on the black beans, salsa, and avocado. Season with salt and pepper, if using, and garnish with cilantro and lime.

Enjoy your yummy, healthy meal!

Landlocked Ceviche

<u>Ingredients Needed</u>

1 small head of cauliflower, finely chopped (about 2½ cups)

2 cups tomatoes, diced (about 4 medium)

½ cup chopped red onion

1 jalapeno, diced

¼ teaspoon salt

½ cup lime juice

¼ cup chopped cilantro

1 avocado, diced

Freshly ground black pepper, to taste

Method

Mix together the cauliflower, tomatoes, red onion, jalapeño, salt, and lime juice in a medium bowl. Add the cilantro and let the mixture sit in the fridge for at least 1 hour.

Add the avocado and black pepper to taste. Serve immediately.

Delicious Black Beans

Ingredients Needed

1 medium onion, small diced

1 red bell pepper, small diced

4 garlic cloves, sliced or diced

2 teaspoons salt

3 teaspoons cumin

3 teaspoons minced oregano

½ to 1 teaspoon red wine vinegar

Two 14-ounce cans black beans, with liquid

¼ to ½ cup water or Vegetable Stock

Method

Heat a medium pot over medium heat. Add the onion and bell pepper and cook until the onion is translucent, stirring occasionally. Add water 1 to 2 tablespoons at a time as needed, to keep the vegetables from sticking to the pan.

Mix in the garlic, salt, cumin, and oregano, and cook for another minute or so. Stir in a splash of red wine vinegar.

Add the beans and water or Vegetable Stock and simmer over medium to medium-low heat for 8 to 10 minutes, until it reaches your desired consistency. (As long as you cook down the pepper and onion in the beginning, there really is no right or wrong amount of time to cook your beans. Taste them along the way and see what texture and consistency you prefer. They can look a bit unappealing when they're broken down after being cooked for a long time, but, man, are they delicious!)

Enjoy with tortillas, rice, or potatoes and serve with garnishes of your choice.

French Green Lentil Salad

Ingredients Needed

FOR THE LENTILS

3 cups dried French green lentils, rinsed and drained

5 cups water

2 teaspoons reduced sodium vegetable broth

4 stalks celery, diced (about 1½ cups)

1½ cups cherry tomatoes, halved

2 medium shallots, finely diced (or ½ small onion)

¼ cup packed chopped fresh parsley

Pinch of sea salt (optional)

FOR THE DRESSING

2 teaspoons Dijon mustard

2 tablespoons red wine vinegar

1 teaspoon herbes de Provence

Freshly ground black pepper, to taste

1 medium clove garlic, minced

Method

To make the lentils, combine the lentils, water, and broth in a saucepan and bring to a boil over high heat. Reduce the heat to medium-low, cover, and simmer for 15 to 20 minutes, until the lentils are tender but firm.

Remove from the heat, drain any remaining liquid, and transfer the lentils to a large bowl. Chill in the refrigerator for at least 30 minutes.

Stir in the celery, tomatoes, shallots, and parsley.

To make the dressing, combine the mustard, vinegar, herbes de Provence, pepper, and garlic in a small dish, and whisk.

Pour the dressing over the lentil mixture and toss well to combine. Season with salt to taste, if desired. Serve chilled.

Easy Vegan Baked Beans

<u>Ingredients Needed</u>

2 (15-ounce) cans pinto beans, rinsed and drained

2 cups Del's Basic Barbecue Sauce

<u>Method</u>

Preheat the oven to 325°F.

Combine the pinto beans and barbecue sauce in a large bowl, and mix well. Transfer the beans to an 8 × 8-inch casserole dish.

Bake, uncovered, for 1 hour. Let stand for 5 minutes before serving.

Black Bean and Sweet Potato Hash

<u>Ingredients Needed</u>

1 cup chopped onion

1 to 2 cloves garlic, minced

2 cups chopped peeled sweet potatoes (about 2 small or medium)

2 teaspoons mild or hot chili powder

⅓ cup low-sodium vegetable broth

1 cup cooked black beans

¼ cup chopped scallions

Splash of hot sauce (optional)

Chopped cilantro, for garnish

Sliced avocado, for garnish (optional)

Oil-free whole wheat or corn tortillas, for serving (optional)

Method

Stovetop Method

1. Place the onions in a nonstick skillet and sauté over medium- heat, stirring occasionally, for 2 to 3 minutes. Add the garlic and stir.

2. Add the sweet potatoes and chili powder, and stir to coat the vegetables with the chili powder. Add broth and stir. Cook for about 12 minutes more, stirring occasionally, until the potatoes are

cooked through. Add more liquid 1 to 2 tablespoons at a time as needed, to keep the vegetables from sticking to the pan.

3. Add the black beans, scallions, and salt. Cook for 1 or 2 minutes more, until the beans are heated through.

4. Add the hot sauce (if using), and stir. Taste and adjust the seasonings. Top with chopped cilantro and serve.

Pressure Cooker Method

1. Heat a stovetop pressure cooker over medium heat or set an electric cooker to sauté. Add the onion and cook, stirring occasionally, for 2 to 3 minutes. Add the garlic and stir. Add the sweet potatoes and chili powder. Stir to coat the sweet potatoes with the chili powder. Add the broth and stir.

2. Lock the lid on the pressure cooker. Bring to high pressure for 3 minutes. Quick release the pressure. Remove the lid, tilting it away from you.

3. Add the black beans, scallions, and salt. Cook for 1 or 2 minutes more over medium heat, or lock on

the lid for 3 minutes, until the beans are heated through.

4. Add the hot sauce (if using), and stir. Taste and adjust the seasonings. Top with chopped cilantro and serve.

Asian Cucumber and Sea Vegetable Salad

Ingredients Needed

FOR THE DRESSING

3 tablespoons brown rice vinegar

2 tablespoons freshly squeezed lemon juice

Zest of 1 lemon

1 tablespoon evaporated cane sugar

1 tablespoon pickled ginger, finely chopped

1 teaspoon dried minced onion

½ teaspoon sea salt

2 teaspoons sesame seeds, plus more for garnish

FOR THE SALAD

¼ cup dried wakame seaweed

2 hothouse cucumbers, cut into ¼-inch-thick rounds

½ cup shredded carrots

Method

To prepare the dressing, whisk vinegar, lemon juice and zest, sugar, ginger, dried onion, sea salt, and 2 teaspoons sesame seeds together in a small bowl. Set aside.

To prepare the salad, soak wakame in warm water for 3 to 5 minutes to rehydrate. Drain and chop, if desired. Place in large serving bowl. Add cucumbers and carrots.

Add dressing to vegetables and toss. Serve right away, garnished with additional sesame seeds.

Quinoa Primavera

Ingredients Needed

CITRUS-PICKLED SHALLOTS

2 large shallots, cut into half-moons

2 tablespoons orange juice

½ teaspoon apple cider vinegar

½ teaspoon salt

Pinch of sugar

QUINOA

Ingredients Needed

1 cup quinoa, soaked at least 2 hours or overnight, rinsed, and drained

2 cups frozen artichoke hearts (see note)

2 garlic cloves, minced

1 teaspoon dried tarragon

½ teaspoon dried thyme

½ teaspoon salt, plus more to taste

¼ teaspoon dried dill

¼ teaspoon black pepper, plus more to taste

2 cups frozen peas

2 carrots, diced

1 orange or yellow bell pepper, finely chopped

3 scallions (white and light green parts), thinly sliced

zest and juice of 1 lemon

½ cup raw sunflower seeds

Method

To make the shallots, combine all the Ingredients Needed in a small bowl. Refrigerate until ready to serve. (The shallots can be refrigerated overnight or up to 3 days.)

To make the quinoa, combine 2 cups water and quinoa in a large saucepan over high heat. Bring to a boil, then add the artichokes, garlic, tarragon, thyme, ½ teaspoon salt, the dill, and ¼ teaspoon pepper. Reduce the heat to medium-low, cover, and cook for 10 minutes. Reduce the heat to low and stir in the peas, carrots, bell pepper, and scallions. Cover and cook until the vegetables are heated through, about 5 minutes.

Remove from the heat, add the lemon juice and zest and the sunflower seeds, fluff with a fork, and season with salt and pepper. Serve, topping each portion with the shallots.

DELECTABLE LUNCH IDEAS

Irish White Bean and Cabbage Stew

Ingredients Needed

1 large onion, chopped

3 ribs celery, chopped

2 to 3 cloves garlic, minced

½ head cabbage, chopped

4 carrots, sliced

1 to 1-½ pounds potatoes, cut in large dice

1 bay leaf

1 teaspoon dried thyme

½ teaspoon caraway seeds

½ teaspoon dried rosemary, crushed

½ teaspoon freshly ground black pepper

⅓ cup pearled barley (optional or substitute with gluten-free grain)

6-8 cups vegetable broth or low-sodium vegetable broth

3 cups cooked great northern beans (2 cans, drained)

1 14 ½-ounce can diced tomatoes

1 tablespoon chopped fresh parsley

salt to taste

<u>Method</u>

Crock Pot: Place the vegetables, seasonings, and barley into a large (at least 5 quart) slow cooker. Add enough vegetable broth to just cover the vegetables (start with 6 cups and add more as needed). Cover and cook on low heat for 7 hours. Add beans, tomatoes, parsley, and salt to taste. Check seasonings and add more herbs if necessary. Cover and cook for another hour.

Stovetop: Place vegetables, seasonings, barley, and broth into a large stockpot. Cover and simmer until vegetables are tender, about 45 minutes. Add beans, tomatoes, parsley, and salt to taste. Check seasonings and add more herbs if necessary. Simmer uncovered for at least 15 minutes before serving.

Fettuccine with Grilled Asparagus, Peas, and Lemon

Ingredients Needed

6-8 stalks asparagus

2 cloves garlic, minced

Juice of 1 lemon, about 2 tablespoons

Pinch of coarse sea salt

Water

6 ounces fettuccine

2 tablespoons minced parsley

1 cup fresh or frozen peas

Method

Toss the asparagus in the garlic, lemon juice, and salt.

Grill the asparagus until it just starts to develop a few blackened spots. The asparagus should still have some crispness to it.

Cut the asparagus into 2-inch pieces.

Bring the water to a boil. Add the pasta and boil until it pasta is al dente, adding peas to the pot during the last minutes of cooking.

Drain the pasta and peas and return to pot. Add the asparagus and parsley, and toss to combine.

Italian White Bean, Kale and Potato Stew

<u>Ingredients Needed</u>

1 cup diced red or white onion

3 cloves garlic

2 28 ounce cans diced tomatoes (salt free if you prefer)

¼ - ½ teaspoon red pepper flakes

5 cups red-skinned potatoes cut into one inch squares

1 tablespoon dried oregano

1 tablespoon dried parsley

6-8 packed cups of kale, after it has been de-stemmed and chopped

2 15 ounce cans Cannellini beans, drained and rinsed

salt (optional)

<u>Method</u>

Place a large soup/stock pot over a medium high flame and pour some of the liquid from one of the cans of the diced tomatoes into the pot to cover the base of the pot. When the tomato liquid starts to bubble, add the onion and stir. Lower heat a little. Press garlic into pot. Add red pepper flakes (to taste). Continue to cook and stir, lowering heat as the time passes, for a total of about 10 minutes or until onions are soft.

Add the rest of the first can of diced tomatoes and the entire second can into the pot. Bring heat up to medium-high again so that tomatoes begin to simmer. Place diced potatoes, oregano and parsley into the pot and stir. Cover pot, lower heat to low and simmer for 20 minutes.

Place all of the kale into the pot and cover the pot again. Let kale steam and shrink for 3 minutes. Uncover pot and stir in kale. Add Cannellini beans and stir. Taste and season with salt (or not). If potatoes are not as soft as you desire, continue to let simmer.

Herbed Hummus

<u>Ingredients Needed</u>

1 cup fresh basil leaves, lightly packed and blanched

½ cup fresh tarragon leaves, lightly packed and blanched

4 cups cooked garbanzo beans

1 cup vegetable broth

½ cup fresh flat-leaf parsley leaves, lightly packed

Juice of 1 lemon

2 tablespoons sesame seeds, toasted

2 cloves garlic

¼ cup chopped chives

<u>Method</u>

Pat the basil and tarragon dry and coarsely chop them. Transfer to a food processor. Add the beans, broth, parsley, lemon juice, sesame seeds, and garlic and process until the desired consistency is achieved. Stir in the chives. Stored in a sealed container in the refrigerator, Herbed Hummus will keep for 4 days.

Note: Most food processors don't do a good job of chopping chives, as the chives tend to get wound around the base of the blade. That's why I suggest you chop them by hand.

Veggie Wraps with Herbed Hummus

Ingredients Needed

12 to 16 collard green leaves, stemmed

1 cucumber, peeled and cut into thin strips

1 red bell pepper, cut into thin strips

½ medium jicama, peeled and cut into thin strips

½ cup hearts of palm, cut into strips, rinsed, and patted dry

1 small carrot, peeled and cut into thin strips

1 stalk celery, cut into thin strips

2 cups Herbed Hummus

1 ripe avocado, sliced

½ cup cashews, toasted and slightly crushed

20 fresh basil leaves

1 tablespoon chopped fresh chives

Method

Steam the collard green leaves for 1 minute. Remove immediately and let cool. Lay flat and arrange into four 8 x 10-inch rectangles. Lay a paper towel on top of each rectangle and roll a rolling pin over the leaves to crush the veins.

Put the cucumber, bell pepper, jicama, hearts of palm, carrot, and celery in a medium bowl and stir until well combined.

To assemble a wrap, put a rectangle of collard green leaves on a cutting board and spread one-quarter of the hummus along one of the longer edges, then arrange one-quarter of the avocado on top of the hummus and one quarter of the cucumber mixture, cashews, basil, and chives alongside the hummus. Roll up halfway, tucking in the ends so the filling won't squeeze out. Finish by rolling the wrap as tightly as possible. Assemble the remaining wraps in the same fashion (to make 4 wraps in all).

Serve the wraps whole and eat them like burritos, or cut them into slices and serve them on a plate like sushi. Veggie Wraps with Herbed Hummus can be assembled in advance. Individually wrapped in plastic and stored in the refrigerator, they will keep for 2 days.

Curried French Lentils

Ingredients Needed

6 cups water

1 cup French Green lentils

1 yellow onion, chopped

1 small yam or sweet potato, diced (about two cups)

2 cups small cauliflower florets

2 ribs celery, sliced

1 can (14.5-ounce) diced, salt-free tomatoes

2 teaspoons curry powder

2 teaspoons dried green herbs (like a French or Italian blend)

1 teaspoon granulated onion

1 teaspoon granulated garlic

4 cups greens cut into bite-size pieces (like kale, chard, spinach, collards, beet greens)

Method

In a soup pot on high, bring the water and lentils to a boil. Reduce heat to medium and cook for 20 minutes (a low boil).

Add the onion, yam/sweet potato, cauliflower, celery, tomatoes (including juice), and the four herbs and spices. Cook for 10 minutes at the same heat. Add greens, and cook for 5-10 more minutes (spinach, chard and beet greens won't take as long to cook as kale or collard greens), until potatoes and greens are tender. Serve as is or over cooked brown rice.

Notes:

Soup, stew or filling: As written, this recipe is more of a stew than a soup (especially upon reheating the next day), so I like to serve it over brown or wild rice, or in a corn tortilla with a little avocado on top. But you can easily make it into a soup by adding 1-2 cups of water in step two.

Lentils: A variety of lentils exist, and can be used in this recipe by adjusting the cooking time slightly (mainly for red lentils, which take only 25-30 minutes to cook).

Tomatoes: Fresh tomatoes can also be used, especially when they are in season (about 1-½ cups diced).

Broccoli option: If you're not a fan of cauliflower, broccoli may be used (or both).

Black Bean and Sweet Potato Soup

Ingredients Needed

1-2 tablespoon(s) water

1½ - 1¾ cups chopped onions (one large onion)

1½ cups combination of chopped red peppers and green peppers

1¼ teaspoon sea salt

freshly ground black pepper to taste (generous is good)

2 teaspoons cumin seeds

2 teaspoons dried oregano leaves

¼ teaspoon allspice (rounded)

¼ teaspoon (or less/more, to taste) red pepper flakes

4 medium-large cloves garlic, minced or grated

4½ - 5 cups black beans (reserve 1 cup; drain and rinse if using canned - about three 14 or 15 ounce cans)

3 cups water

2 tablespoons tomato paste

1 tablespoon balsamic vinegar

2 tablespoons freshly squeezed lime juice

½ - 1 teaspoon pure maple syrup

1 bay leaf

1½ cups cubed (in small chunks, about ½") yellow sweet potato (or can substitute white potato)

Chopped cilantro for serving

Extra lime wedges for serving

Chopped avocado tossed with lemon juice and dash of salt, for serving

Method

In a large pot over medium-high heat, add water, onions, red and green peppers, salt and pepper, cumin seeds, oregano, allspice, and red pepper flakes. Let cook for 5-7 minutes until onions and peppers start to soften.

Add garlic. Cover, reduce heat to medium, and let cook another few minutes to soften garlic - if sticking/burning, add another splash of water.

After a few minutes of cooking, add 3½ cups beans (reserving one cup of beans), water, tomato paste, vinegar, lime juice, and maple syrup (start with ½ teaspoon).

Using an immersion blender, puree soup until fairly smooth.

Increase heat to bring to boil, add bay leaf and diced sweet potatoes, then once at boil reduce and let simmer for 20-30 minutes.

Add remaining cup of black beans and extra maple syrup if desired (taste test). Stir through, let simmer for another few minutes, then serve, topping with cilantro if desired and with lime wedges. Also delicious to top soup with some chopped seasoned avocado or a simple guacamole.

Sweet Potato Tip: Sometimes I have leftover sweet potato home fries that have been seasoned with just sea salt. If so, I take a recipe and chopping shortcut and simply add these to my soup during the last 5-10 minutes of cooking, just to heat through

Boulangere Potatoes

<u>Ingredients Needed</u>

1 leek, thinly sliced

1 yellow onion, thinly sliced

1 stalk celery, thinly sliced

2 shallots, thinly sliced

2 tablespoons chopped garlic

1 tablespoon granulated garlic

1 tablespoon granulated onion

6 cups low-sodium vegetable broth

9 medium Yukon gold potatoes, peeled and very
thinly sliced

1 tablespoon chopped, fresh flat-leaf parsley, or 1
teaspoon dried

1 tablespoon chopped fresh thyme, or 1 teaspoon
dried

Method

Preheat the oven to 350º F. Put the leek, onion,
celery, shallots, and garlic in a large dry saucepan
over medium heat and cook, stirring constantly,
until the onion starts to brown, about 5 minutes.

Stir in the granulated garlic and granulated onion and cook for 2 minutes. Stir in the broth, increase the heat to medium-high, and simmer until the liquid is reduced by half.

Add the potatoes and stir until well combined. Decrease the heat to low and cook, stirring constantly so the potatoes don't stick together, until the potatoes are translucent, about 15 minutes.

Remove from the heat and stir in the parsley and thyme. Transfer to 13x9-inch baking dish and bake uncovered for about 25 minutes, until the potatoes are golden brown and fork-tender. Serve hot.

Navy Bean Soup

<u>**Ingredients Needed**</u>

1 bay leaf

1 cup celery, diced

1 onion, diced

2 carrots, diced

2 cups cooked navy beans

Low-sodium vegetable broth

½ teaspoon salt, or to taste

1 teaspoon oregano

1 tablespoon sweet white miso, diluted in ¼ cup water

2 cups chopped kale

Method

In a large soup pot, layer the bay leaf, celery, onion and carrots. Add the beans on top. Cover with the vegetable broth and bring to a boil.

Cover the pot and reduce the heat to simmer on low for 30 minutes or until the vegetables are tender.

Add the salt, oregano, miso and kale. Simmer for 10 minutes. Adjust seasonings to taste. *Optional: Before adding the kale, puree half of the soup in a blender for a thicker consistency.

Greek Stuffed Peppers

<u>Ingredients Needed</u>

6 large or 8 small bell peppers

1 large onion, diced

3 small zucchini, peeled and diced

3 medium carrots, peeled and diced

1 cup low-sodium vegetable broth

3 cups cooked brown rice

5 tablespoons tomato paste

¾ cup fresh parsley, chopped

¾ cup fresh dill, chopped

1 lemon, juiced

¼ teaspoon pepper

½ teaspoon Herbamare or salt

Method

Preheat oven to 350º F.

Cut around stem of peppers like you would cut a jack-o-lantern top, retaining the top with stem. Remove seeds carefully and wash and dry thoroughly.

Place peppers in an oven safe dish and arrange upright and put tops back on.

Bake at 350º F for 30 minutes.

Meanwhile in a large non stick pan, saute onions, zucchini and carrots in vegetable broth for 5-6 minutes.

Stir in the rice and tomato paste and coat thoroughly.

Add parsley, dill, lemon juice, pepper and Herbamare (or salt) and stir to combine.

When peppers are ready, take out of oven and fill with stuffing.

Place tops back on peppers and bake for an extra 30-40 minutes until the peppers are soft.

Serve with additional wedges of lemon and dill for garnish if desired.

Vegan Pasta Primavera

<u>**Ingredients Needed**</u>

12 ounces quinoa penne

3 cups broccoli, chopped

2 cups carrots, diced

1 onion, diced

1 cup red bell pepper, diced

1½ tablespoon garlic granules

2 cups low-sodium vegetable broth

½ cup raw cashews

1 cup soy milk

½ cup oat flour

2 cups green peas

¼ teaspoon black pepper

2 teaspoons dried basil or 2 tablespoons fresh

2 teaspoons dried oregano or 2 tablespoons fresh

1 cup cherry tomatoes, halved

Method

In a medium pot, bring water to a boil. Then add the pasta and cook according to the directions on the box. When the pasta is slightly al dente, remove from heat, drain, and set aside. While pasta cooks, in a large sauté pan, sweat (see chef's note below) the broccoli, carrots, onion, red pepper, and garlic on medium heat for 10 minutes.

Keep them covered and stir occasionally. Then stir in the vegetable broth and simmer for another 10 minutes.

Grind the cashews in a spice grinder to form a cashew powder. A coffee grinder or blender would also work. Either way, make sure the appliance is completely dry.

Stir in the soy milk, oat flour and cashew powder. Make sure to stir occasionally to prevent the oats from clumping together. Add the peas, black pepper, and dried herbs. Simmer for 10 minutes, continuing to stir occasionally, until the oats and cashews create a creamy sauce. Mix in the pasta and tomatoes. Best served right away. Also delicious chilled as a pasta salad.

Sweating is a mix of sautéing and steaming. The idea is the water will come out or "sweat" from the veggies, which creates enough moisture so that no added liquid is needed. To sweat an item, put the cut veggie in a sauté pan without oil or water over medium heat. Keep the pan covered and stir frequently. Do this until the item is cooked to desired frequency. If the pan is becoming dry or veggie starts to stick to the bottom of pan, add a little bit of water or vegetable broth. You can also turn down the heat.

Because you are grinding the cashews and using oat flour, they will be slightly coarse and you will likely see specks of these two within the cream sauce. If this bothers you, you could try substituting a more refined thickening agent, such as store-bought rice flour or potato starch.

If you are using fresh herbs, add them in the last step when you are mixing in the pasta and tomatoes.

Macadamia-Vanilla Frosting

Ingredients Needed

½ cup macadamia nuts, soaked in ½ cup water for 15 to 30 minutes

6 medjool dates, pitted and diced, soaked in ½ cup water for 15 to 30 minutes

1 teaspoon vanilla extract

<u>Method</u>

Drain the soaked nuts and discard the water.

Add all Ingredients Needed (the nuts, dates with their soak water, and vanilla) to a blender, and purée until smooth and even in color.

Add a little more water as needed, to keep the blender moving if the mixture gets too thick.

Fast Pizza

<u>Ingredients Needed</u>

PIZZA BASE

1 pita bread

¼ cup low-sodium tomato sauce

⅛ teaspoon dried basil

⅛ teaspoon dried oregano

TOPPINGS

⅛ cup chopped yellow onions

⅛ cup chopped scallions

⅛ cup chopped green peppers

4 sliced mushrooms

⅛ cup alfalfa sprouts

Method

Cut the pita bread in half by separating it into two circles. Spread each half with tomato sauce.

Sprinkle on the basil and oregano and add the toppings of your choice.

Bake at 300º F for 10 minutes, or heat in toaster oven for 5 minutes at 250ºF.

Trumpet Vegan Sushi Rolls

Ingredients Needed

2 cups sweet brown rice

4 cups water

4-6 Trumpet mushrooms

1 teaspoon garlic powder

1 teaspoon granulated onion

½-1 cup water for sauteing

2 large carrots, julienned

1 cucumber, seeded and julienned

2 avocados, sliced

20 leaves fresh basil, chopped

4-6 sheets of sushi nori (made from seaweed)

Method

Combine the rice and water in a large pan, bring to a boil, reduce heat to simmer and cover. Cook for 50 minutes. Remove from heat and let stand with lid on for 10 minutes. Remove lid, set aside and let cool. While the rice is cooking, prepare the mushrooms and filling Ingredients Needed.

To prepare the Trumpet mushrooms, cut them into lengths and sauté them with the onion and garlic powder, adding water as you go so they do not stick. Sauté for 5 to 10 minutes until softened. Remove and set aside.

Using a mandolin slicer, julienne the carrots and cucumber; or use a chef's knife to cut into very thin strips. Slice the avocado after removing the skin and pit. Chop the basil. Put everything on a big plate (in piles) so you'll be ready to roll (so to speak) with your nori sheets.

Place a piece of Nori on top of a sushi mat (or silicone mat or a 12×12-inch square of plastic wrap), and spread about a half-cup of rice in a thin layer over most of the seaweed wrapper, leaving some space around the edges. Arrange the mushrooms and vegetables in a line parallel to the bottom edge (closest to you). You can put in as much or little as you like.

To roll up, follow the directions on the nori package, or simply roll away from you, keeping the Ingredients Needed tight together so they don't spill out on the sides or front (you should be rolling with the sushi mat too; this keeps things even and helps the nori not to tear). After the first complete roll, squeeze it in toward you to really smash everything together (this will keep things from falling out after you cut the roll). Continue to roll again so that the remaining bit of nori is rolled up and it looks like one long tube. Give it another really firm squeeze. Remove it from the sushi mat and, using a serrated knife, cut into two large pieces, or four to six smaller pieces (you may want to trim off the ends).

Optional: Garnish with sesame seeds. If you want to use soy sauce or tamari (fermented, wheat-free soy sauce), you can dilute it with water to lower the sodium content. I also like to use a little wasabi (a flavor between hot mustard and horseradish). Sometimes I make a dipping sauce in my high-speed blender, using 8 soaked macadamia nuts (other nuts would work too), ½ teaspoon of wasabi powder, 4 tablespoons of water and a little fresh ginger.

Mushrooms: Trumpet mushrooms are so great in this, but you may also use any other kind of mushroom. Shitakes would be my second choice due to their chewy texture, but portabella and cremini would be good too.

Rice: I like using "sweet brown" rice for these rolls because it is the stickiest of the brown rices (like sushi rice). You may also use regular "short-grain" brown rice, Lundberg's "Golden Rose" brown rice, or "Haiga" rice (partially milled with the bran removed but not the germ). Haiga is a little harder to find in regular stores, but I have found it at Whole Foods in the bulk section, or at Asian markets (its shape and color is closest to white rice).

You may also use lightly steamed cauliflower instead of brown rice, but don't over-steam it because it will get too mushy. Pulse the cauliflower a few times in the food processor until it looks like rice; don't over-pulse. While I'm not a fan of the strong flavor, some people like to use the cauliflower raw (but still pulsed in the food processer).

Rice seasoning: In traditional sushi roll recipes, the rice is seasoned with rice vinegar, salt, sugar and/or mirin, a sweet Japanese rice wine. I have skipped this step because I think it tastes just fine without these additions, and it also cuts out a step (and I don't use salt or sugar in my recipes). But if you want to go the traditional route, just Google "sushi rice" recipes.

Collards instead of Nori: You may also use steamed collard greens instead of nori seaweed sheets. Just trim the thick ends of the collards, steam or boil them for 5 or so minutes (they are pretty sturdy), and blot off water with a paper towel. Let cool before filling. Roll as usual, but after first roll and squeeze, tuck the ends in (like a spring roll), then finish rolling. You could use the collards raw, but they are very fibrous and can be hard to chew.

Optional filling items: Sprouts, bell peppers, Daikon radish, scallions, tofu, cilantro, pea shoots, peanuts or walnuts, cooked soba noodles (cold).

Autumn Minestrone

Ingredients Needed

1 medium onion, cut into ½-inch pieces

2 stalks celery, sliced crosswise into ½-inch pieces

½ bulb fennel, cut into 1-by-¼-inch pieces (about 1½ cups)

2 medium Yukon gold potatoes, peeled and cut into 1-inch pieces

2-3 cloves garlic, finely chopped

1 can (35 ounces) whole tomatoes, lightly crushed

8 cups low-sodium vegetable broth

1 can (15 ounces) cannellini beans, drained and rinsed

Salt and pepper, to taste

2 teaspoons red-wine vinegar

1 zucchini, quartered and sliced

1½ bunches Swiss chard leaves, thinly sliced (about 6 cups)

2 cups cooked elbow or fusilli pasta (eggless)

Nutritional yeast or finely ground pumpkin seeds for garnish

Method

Heat enough water that fills the bottom of the pan in an 8-quart stockpot over medium high heat. Add onion, celery, fennel, potatoes, and garlic and cook, stirring occasionally, about 5 minutes.

Add tomatoes and their juices, stock, and cannellini beans; season with 2 teaspoons salt and ½ teaspoon pepper. Increase heat to high and bring to a boil. Reduce heat to a simmer, add in the zucchini and cook until potatoes are tender, about 10 minutes.

Stir in vinegar and Swiss chard; season with salt and pepper. Divide pasta evenly between 6 to 8 bowls. Ladle over soup and garnish with nutritional yeast or ground pumpkin seeds. Serve immediately and enjoy!

Lentil Shepherd's Pie with Rustic Parsnip Crust

Ingredients Needed

1 large yellow onion, peeled and diced small

1 large carrot, peeled and diced small

2 stalks celery, diced small

2 cloves garlic, peeled and minced

1 sprig rosemary

1½ cup green lentils, rinsed

1 bay leaf

3 tablespoons tomato paste

Salt and freshly ground black pepper to taste

8 medium red-skin potatoes, peeled and chopped

4 parsnips, peeled and chopped

Method

Place the onion, carrot, and celery in a large saucepan and sauté over medium heat for 10 minutes. Add water 1 to 2 tablespoons at a time to keep the vegetables from sticking to the pan. Add the garlic and cook for another minute. Stir in the rosemary, lentils, bay leaf, and enough water to cover the lentils by 3 inches. Bring the pot to a boil over high heat. Reduce the heat to medium and cook, covered, for 30 minutes.

Preheat the oven to 350° F.

Add the tomato paste to the saucepan and cook for another 15 minutes, or until the lentils are tender. Season with salt and pepper. Remove from the heat, discard the bay leaf and rosemary sprig, and pour the lentils into a 9 × 13-inch baking dish.

Meanwhile, add the potatoes and parsnips to a medium saucepan and add enough water to cover. Bring the pot to a boil over high heat. Reduce the heat to medium and cook, covered, until the vegetables are tender, about 15 minutes.

Remove the potatoes and parsnips from the heat and drain all but ½ cup of the water. Mash the vegetables until smooth and creamy, then season with additional salt and spread the mixture evenly over the lentils.

Bake the casserole for 25 minutes, or until bubbly. Let sit for 10 minutes before serving.

DELECTABLE DINNER RECIPE IDEAS

Zucchini, Corn, and Black Bean Soup

Ingredients Needed

1 32-oz. carton unsweetened, unflavored almond milk

2 cups ½-inch pieces peeled russet potatoes

½ cup chopped onion

½ cup chopped celery

2 cloves garlic, minced

2 cups fresh corn

1 15-oz. can no-salt-added black beans, rinsed and drained

1 medium zucchini, quartered lengthwise and cut into ¼-inch slices

1 teaspoon snipped fresh thyme

2 tablespoons sherry vinegar

Sea salt and freshly ground black pepper, to taste

Method

In a 4-qt. Dutch oven combine almond milk, potatoes, onion, celery, and garlic. Bring to boiling; reduce heat. Simmer 10 to 12 minutes or until potatoes are tender, stirring occasionally.

Stir in corn, beans, zucchini, and thyme. Return to boiling; reduce heat. Simmer 10 minutes or until zucchini is tender. Stir in vinegar and season with salt and pepper.

Garden Chickpea Tomato Soup

Ingredients Needed

3 lb. tomatoes, seeded and chopped

1 cup chopped sweet onion, such as Vidalia or Maui

1 cup chopped red bell pepper

3 cloves garlic, chopped

1 15-oz. can no-salt-added chickpeas, rinsed and drained

1 cup low-sodium vegetable broth

Sea salt, to taste

Freshly ground black pepper, to taste

1 cup yellow cherry or grape tomatoes, quartered

¼ cup unsalted raw pumpkin seeds (pepitas), toasted

2 tablespoons snipped fresh parsley

Method

Working in batches, in a food processor or blender combine the first four ingredients (through garlic). Cover and process or blend until smooth.

In a 4-qt. Dutch oven combine pureed vegetables, the chickpeas, and broth. Bring to boiling; reduce heat. Simmer, covered, 10 minutes. Season with salt and pepper.

Top servings with quartered tomatoes, pumpkin seeds, and parsley.

Mediterranean Lentil and Spinach Soup

Ingredients Needed

32 ounces low-sodium vegetable broth

1 cup brown or green lentils, rinsed and drained

1 medium onion, chopped (1 cup)

2 stalks celery, chopped (½ cup)

1 carrot, chopped (½ cup)

3 cloves garlic, minced

1 green zucchini or yellow squash, cut into ½-inch pieces

1 teaspoon ground cumin

1 teaspoon fresh oregano, snipped

2 medium tomatoes, chopped (2 cups)

Sea salt and freshly ground black pepper, to taste

4 cups fresh baby spinach

Method

In a 6-qt. Dutch oven combine the first six ingredients (through garlic) and 1 cup water. Bring to boiling over medium-high; reduce heat. Simmer, covered, 25 to 30 minutes or just until lentils are tender.

Stir in squash, cumin, and oregano. Simmer, uncovered, 10 minutes more or until squash is tender. Stir in tomatoes; heat through. Season with salt and pepper. Remove from heat. Before serving, stir in spinach.

30-Minute Chili

Ingredients Needed

2 yellow onions, chopped (1½ cups)

1 large green bell pepper, chopped (1½ cups)

3 tablespoons mild chili powder

1 tablespoon dried oregano

2 teaspoons ground cumin

4 cloves garlic, minced

2 15-oz. cans pinto beans, rinsed and drained

1 28-oz. can diced tomatoes, undrained

2 cups low-sodium vegetable broth

Sea salt, to taste

Freshly ground black pepper, to taste

Cooked brown rice or whole grain noodles (optional)

<u>Method</u>

In a Dutch oven cook onions and bell peppers over medium 5 minutes or until softened, stirring occasionally and adding water, 1 to 2 Tbsp. at a time, as needed to prevent sticking.

Stir in chili powder, oregano, cumin, and garlic; cook 1 minute. Add beans, tomatoes, and broth. Bring just to boiling over medium-high; reduce heat. Simmer, partially covered, 20 minutes or until tomatoes start to break down and mixture is slightly thick.

Season with salt and black pepper. If desired, serve chili over rice.

Red Curry Noodle Soup

Ingredients Needed

8 oz. dried pad Thai brown rice noodles, broken into 2-inch pieces

2 cups low-sodium vegetable broth

2 tablespoons red curry paste

6 cloves garlic, minced

1 tablespoon finely chopped fresh lemongrass

2 teaspoons grated fresh ginger

1 large red bell pepper, chopped (1 cup)

1 cup bias-sliced fresh snow pea pods

2 carrots, cut or shredded into thin bite-size strips
(1 cup)

2 cups unsweetened coconut milk beverage

Sea salt, to taste

¼ cup thinly sliced fresh basil leaves

¼ cup fresh cilantro leaves

½ onion, very thinly sliced (¼ cup)

1 fresh Fresno, jalapeño, or serrano chile pepper,
thinly sliced (optional)

1 lime, cut into 4 wedges

Method

Cook noodles according to package directions; drain.

Meanwhile, in a 4-qt. Dutch oven combine broth, curry paste, garlic, lemongrass, and ginger. Bring to boiling; reduce heat. Simmer 5 minutes.

Stir in bell pepper, pea pods, and carrots. Return to boiling; reduce heat. Simmer 5 minutes more. Stir in coconut milk and cooked noodles; heat through. Season with salt.

Top servings with basil, cilantro, onion, and, if desired, chile pepper. Serve with lime wedges.

Instant Pot Kidney Bean Dal

Ingredients Needed

1½ cups dried red kidney beans, rinsed and drained

1 large onion chopped (1 cup)

1 medium tomato, coarsely chopped (1 cup)

2 whole pitted dates

3 cloves garlic, minced

1 tablespoon ground coriander

1 tablespoon fresh ginger, grated

1½ teaspoon ground cumin

1½ teaspoon garam masala

1 teaspoon ground turmeric

1 cup plant-based milk, unsweetened, unflavored

2 tablespoons fresh cilantro, finely chopped

1 tablespoon lime juice

½ teaspoon sea salt

2 cups hot cooked brown basmati rice, or quinoa or 2 whole wheat pita rounds

Method

In a 6-qt. Instant Pot multicooker combine the first 10 ingredients (through turmeric). Stir in 3 cups water.

Lock lid in place; set pressure valve to Sealing. Set cooker on Bean setting and cook 45 minutes. Let stand to release pressure naturally (about 20 minutes). Open lid carefully.

Stir in plant-based milk, cilantro, lime juice, and salt. Set cooker on Keep Warm setting and heat, uncovered, 10 minutes or until mixture is thick.

Serve bean mixture over rice or quinoa, or with pita rounds.

Cannellini Bean, Kale, and Orzo Soup

Ingredients Needed

1 medium onion, chopped (1 cup)

2 stalks of celery, chopped (1 cup)

2 carrots, chopped (1 cup)

5 sprigs fresh parsley

2 sprigs fresh thyme

2 bay leaves

3 cloves garlic, minced

½ teaspoon sea salt, plus more for seasoning

1 cup whole wheat orzo pasta

1 15-oz. can no-salt-added cannellini (white kidney) beans, rinsed and drained

1 cup stemmed and chopped kale

1 teaspoon finely snipped fresh oregano

1 lemon

Freshly ground black pepper, to taste

Method

In a 5- to 6-qt. Dutch oven combine the first eight ingredients (through the ½ tsp. salt) and 8 cups water. Bring to boiling; reduce heat. Simmer, covered, 20 minutes.

Stir in orzo. Simmer, covered, 10 minutes more, stirring occasionally. Remove and discard parsley and thyme sprigs and bay leaves. Stir in beans, kale, and oregano. Return to boiling; reduce heat. Simmer, covered, 5 minutes more.

Meanwhile, remove ½ teaspoon zest and squeeze 2 tablespoons juice from lemon. Before serving, stir lemon juice into soup. Season with the remaining salt and the pepper to taste. Top servings with lemon zest.

Zesty White Bean Chili

<u>Ingredients Needed</u>

3 bell peppers (red, orange, and/or green), cored and cut into ½-inch dice (3 cups)

1 medium onion, cut into ¼-inch dice (2 cups)

3 celery stalks, cut into ½-inch dice (1½ cups)

2 medium carrots, roughly chopped into ¼-inch pieces (1 cup)

12 cloves garlic, minced

2 teaspoons ground cumin

2 teaspoons dried oregano

2 (15-ounce) cans diced tomatoes (3 cups)

2 tablespoons salt-free chili powder

2 tablespoons paprika

3 (15-ounce) cans cannellini beans, rinsed and drained (4½ cups)

1 cup fresh or frozen corn

2 tablespoons white wine vinegar

1 tablespoon fresh lemon juice

¼ cup finely chopped fresh cilantro, divided

⅓ teaspoon sea salt

Method

In a large saucepan or pot over medium heat, combine the bell peppers, onion, celery, carrots, garlic, cumin, and oregano. Cook 20 minutes, stirring occasionally. Add water, 1 to 2 tablespoons at a time, as needed to prevent vegetables from sticking to the pan.

Add the tomatoes, chili powder, paprika, and 2 cups water. Bring to a boil over high heat; then reduce heat to a simmer, cover pot, and cook 10 minutes more.

Add the beans, corn, vinegar, lemon juice, half of the cilantro, and the salt. Cook 10 to 15 minutes, or until the vegetables are tender and the chili thickens.

Garnish with remaining cilantro and serve hot.

Creamy Wild Rice Soup

Ingredients Needed

4 cups vegetable stock

1 (8-ounce) package button mushrooms, trimmed and quartered

¾ cup uncooked wild rice, rinsed and drained

½ cup thinly sliced leek (white part only)

4 cloves garlic, minced

1 cup chopped red bell pepper

½ cup chopped carrot

¼ teaspoon sea salt

¼ cup almond flour

¼ cup chickpea flour

1 tablespoon snipped fresh thyme

1 tablespoon white wine vinegar

Method

Combine the stock, mushrooms, wild rice, leek, and garlic in a 5-quart Dutch oven or soup pot. Bring to a boil over high heat; reduce heat to medium-low. Cover and simmer for 45 to 50 minutes or until the rice is tender (kernels will start to pop open). Stir in the bell peppers, carrot, and salt. Cover and simmer for 8 minutes more.

Combine the almond flour and chickpea flour in a small bowl; stir in ¼ cup water. Stir the mixture into the soup. Cook, stirring constantly, for 1 to 2 minutes or until thick and bubbly. Stir in up to ½ cup more water to reach the desired consistency. Stir in the thyme and vinegar.

Hearty Vegetarian Chili

Ingredients Needed

1 pound dried kidney, cranberry, or red beans, soaked overnight and drained

1 (14.5-ounce) can no-salt-added diced tomatoes, undrained

1½ cups chopped carrots

1½ cups chopped celery

1½ cups sliced zucchini

1 cup chopped onion

1 cup chopped green bell pepper

1 cup frozen or canned no-salt-added whole-kernel corn

¾ cup dry steel-cut oats

½ cup tomato paste

2 tablespoons low-sodium tamari or soy sauce

3 cloves garlic, minced

1 tablespoon packed brown sugar

1 tablespoon chili powder

2 teaspoons dried oregano, crushed

2 teaspoons dried cilantro, crushed

1 teaspoon ground cumin

1 teaspoon paprika

1 tablespoon fresh lemon juice

Sea salt

Bottled hot pepper sauce

Toppings such as sliced avocado, chopped scallions, and snipped fresh cilantro (optional)

Method

Place the soaked beans in a 4- to 5-quart Dutch oven. Add 6 cups of water. Bring to a boil over high heat; reduce heat to medium-low. Cover and simmer for 45 minutes, stirring occasionally.

Stir in the diced tomatoes and their juice, carrots, celery, zucchini, onion, bell pepper, corn, oats, tomato paste, tamari, garlic, brown sugar, chili powder, oregano, cilantro, cumin, and paprika. Return to a boil over high heat; reduce heat to medium-low.

Cover and simmer for 45 minutes more or until the vegetables are tender, stirring occasionally. Stir in additional water as needed if the chili becomes too thick.

Stir in the lemon juice and season with salt and hot pepper sauce. Serve with toppings (if using).

Roasted Tomato and Red Pepper Soup

<u>Ingredients Needed</u>

4 large tomatoes, cut into large pieces (5 cups)

3 medium red bell peppers, cut into large pieces (3 cups)

1 medium onion, cut into large wedges

3 cloves garlic

4 ounces uncooked penne, orecchiette, or other short-cut pasta (2 cups cooked)

6 ounces green beans, cut into ½-inch pieces (1 cup)

2 medium carrots, cut into ½-inch dice (1 cup)

1 cup frozen green peas, thawed (5 ounces)

1 tablespoon white wine vinegar

1 teaspoon fresh oregano, finely chopped

½ teaspoon sea salt

⅛ teaspoon freshly ground black pepper

1 cup unsweetened, unflavored plant milk

1 tablespoon fresh parsley, finely chopped

Method

Preheat oven to 425°F. Line a baking sheet with parchment paper.

Place tomatoes, bell peppers, onion, and garlic on the baking sheet. Bake for 20 to 30 minutes.

Meanwhile, bring a pot of water to a boil. Add pasta, green beans, and carrots. Cook according to pasta's package Method. Add peas 2 minutes before pasta is done. Drain pasta and vegetables. Set aside.

Transfer the roasted vegetables to a blender. Add vinegar, oregano, salt, black pepper, and 1 cup water. Blend into a smooth soup.

Transfer blended soup to a pot. Bring to a boil. Add milk, pasta, green beans, and carrots. Cook 3 to 4 minutes, until soup is heated through.

Serve soup hot, garnished with parsley.

Lentil Minestrone

<u>Ingredients Needed</u>

1 small onion, chopped (1 cup)

¾ cup dry brown lentils, rinsed

1 carrot, chopped (½ cup)

1 stalk celery, chopped (½ cup)

3 cloves garlic, minced

4 cups vegetable stock

1 teaspoon dried basil, crushed

1 teaspoon dried oregano, crushed

1 large zucchini, chopped (1¼ cups)

4 ounces uncooked whole-grain elbow macaroni or quinoa

½ cup sun-dried tomatoes (not packed in oil), thinly sliced

4 cups torn fresh kale

1 (14.5-ounce) can crushed tomatoes

¼ teaspoon sea salt

Method

In a 4-quart Dutch oven or soup pot, combine the onion, lentils, carrot, celery, garlic, stock, basil, and oregano. Add 1½ cups water. Bring to a boil over high heat; reduce heat to medium-low. Cover and simmer for 30 minutes.

Stir in the zucchini, macaroni (or quinoa), and sundried tomatoes. Simmer, uncovered, for 3 minutes. Stir in the kale, crushed tomatoes, and salt. Simmer, uncovered, until the macaroni (or quinoa) is cooked, checking package Method for cook time.

CHAPTER NINE: TO SUM UP!

In conclusion, the Daniel Fast diet is much more than a way of eating—it's a journey toward greater health, clarity, and spiritual growth. By focusing on whole, plant-based foods and cutting out processed items, you not only nourish your body but also nurture your mind and spirit.

Following the Daniel Fast can bring about noticeable improvements in your digestion, energy levels, and skin. More importantly, it helps you become more mindful of what you eat and why you eat it. Many people find that this diet helps them reconnect with their faith and values, providing a sense of purpose and clarity that extends beyond physical well-being.

Today, it's easier than ever to embrace the Daniel Fast, thanks to a wide array of resources and recipes that make the transition smooth and enjoyable. This diet encourages you to rethink your food choices and adopt a more conscious, healthful approach to eating.

Whether you're motivated by health concerns, a desire for spiritual renewal, or simply wanting to detoxify and reset, the Daniel Fast offers a meaningful way to achieve these goals. It's a path that can lead to lasting positive changes in your life, fostering a deeper understanding of yourself and your relationship with food. By embarking on this journey, you're setting the stage for a healthier, more vibrant, and more fulfilling life.